# BLADDER CANCER

## A Comprehensive Guide to Understanding and Recovering from Bladder Cancer

**CARL JUAN**

# Table of Contents

## Introductory

Bladder cancer develops in the bladder, a pear-shaped hollow organ in the belly button. The kidneys create urine, which is then stored in the bladder until it is expelled from the body. Bladder cancer develops when cells in the bladder lining mutate and multiply uncontrolled, resulting in a tumor.

• Urothelial carcinoma, formerly known as transitional cell carcinoma, is the most frequent form of bladder cancer. Urothelial carcinoma develops in the urothelium, the inner lining of the bladder, but other less common kinds of bladder cancer can also arise, such as squamous cell carcinoma and adenocarcinoma.

The exact reasons why some people get bladder cancer aren't always obvious, although there are certain known risk factors. Among these potential dangers are:

1. **Smoking:** Smoking is one of the most major risk factors for bladder cancer. Tobacco smoke contains a variety of chemicals, some of which can pass through the kidneys' filtering system and into the bladder, where they may have an adverse effect.

**2.** A higher risk of developing bladder cancer has been linked to exposure to chemicals, such as those used in the dye industry, rubber production, and some herbicides.

**3.** The risk of developing bladder cancer increases with age, making elderly people disproportionately affected.

**4.** Bladder cancer is more common in men than in women.

**5.** Recurrent UTIs or prolonged use of a urinary catheter can raise the likelihood of developing chronic bladder infections or irritations.

Blood in the urine (hematuria), urinating frequently, soreness or discomfort while urinating, and back pain are all possible indications of bladder cancer. The prognosis can be improved via early discovery and treatment, therefore anyone experiencing these symptoms should consult a doctor right away.

Depending on the stage and kind of cancer, treatment for bladder cancer may include a mix of surgery, radiation therapy, chemotherapy, immunotherapy, and targeted therapy. Professional medical staff tailor each patient's treatment to their unique needs and the severity of their illness.

If you suspect or have been diagnosed with bladder cancer, it is crucial that you see a doctor to get an accurate diagnosis and learn about your treatment options.

# CHAPTER ONE
## Bladder Cancer: The Fundamentals

Cancer of the bladder develops in the smooth muscle lining of the hollow organ found in the lower abdomen. In order to grasp the fundamentals of bladder cancer, one must be familiar with its essential features:

## 1. Cancer of the Bladder Subtypes:

• The most frequent form of cancer in men is urothelial carcinoma, also known as transitional cell carcinoma. The bladder's inner lining (urothelium) is the point of origin.

• Cancer of the bladder of the squamous cell variety develops in the bladder's lining as a result of long-term irritation or inflammation.

• Adenocarcinoma is a less common type of bladder cancer that develops in the glandular cells that line the bladder.

## 2. Causal Variables:

• Smoking cigarettes exposes the bladder to carcinogenic substances in the bloodstream, making it a major risk factor for bladder cancer.

• Exposure to chemicals at work: positions in the dye industry or rubber production, for example, can raise the risk.

• Most occurrences of bladder cancer are seen in adults over the age of 55, therefore being older is a risk factor.

• **Gender:** Men are at greater risk than women for developing bladder cancer.

Repeated urinary tract infections, long-term catheter use, and exposure to certain medicines all raise the risk of chronic bladder irritation.

## 3. Symptoms:

• Hematuria is the most common sign, and it manifests itself most obviously as pink, red, or brown urine due to the presence of blood.

• Frequent Urination: People with bladder cancer generally suffer increased urgency and frequency in urination.

It's possible to experience pain or burning when urinating.

Pain in the lower back or pelvic region may be a symptom of an advanced case of bladder cancer.

## 4. Diagnosis:

- If blood or abnormal cells are present in the urine, a basic urinalysis will show it.

- Cystoscopy involves inserting a thin, flexible tube equipped with a camera into the bladder to view its inside.

The biopsy procedure can be performed during a cystoscopy.

CT scans, MRI, or ultrasound may be utilized for imaging to ascertain how far along the cancer has progressed.

**5.** Bladder cancer is staged according to how far the disease has gone within the bladder and whether or not it has spread to lymph nodes or other organs in the vicinity. Stages begin at 0 (carcinoma in situ, localized to the lining) and progress to IV (extensive tissue invasion and distant metastasis).

## 6. Treatment:

• The stage and kind of bladder cancer determine the treatment choices available. Common therapies include immunotherapy, targeted therapy, radiation therapy, chemotherapy, and surgery.

• The healthcare team will decide on the best course of treatment, which may include more than one of these methods.

If you have symptoms or risk factors for bladder cancer, you should consult a doctor right once. Better results and a greater likelihood of recovery are possible when the disease is detected and treated early. A patient's treatment plan should be developed in close collaboration with their healthcare providers.

## Factors and Causes

Like many other cancers, the precise cause of bladder cancer is unknown. Genetic, environmental, and behavioral variables all have a role in its onset and progression. Bladder cancer has many potential causes and risk factors, including:

**1. Tobacco use:** Cigarette smoking is the single most important cause of bladder cancer. Cigarette smoke carries toxic compounds that are taken into the bloodstream and released by the kidneys into the urine, exposing the bladder to carcinogens. The risk of developing bladder cancer among smokers is significantly higher than among non-smokers.

**2.** A higher risk of developing bladder cancer has been associated with exposure to certain chemicals and compounds commonly used in the workplace. Aromatic amines, polycyclic aromatic hydrocarbons, and industrial dyes are among substances that may put workers at a higher risk.

**3.** Exposure to chemicals: Arsenic in drinking water is one example of a chemical that, if consumed regularly, can raise the chance of developing bladder cancer.

**4.** Increased risk of bladder cancer has been linked to chronic bladder irritation, which can occur as a result of frequent bladder infections or the use of a urinary catheter for an extended period of time.

**5.** The risk of developing bladder cancer rises with age, hence older persons are disproportionately affected. People over the age of 55 make up the vast bulk of sufferers.

**6.** Approximately three to four times as many men as women will be diagnosed with bladder cancer during their lifetimes.

**7.** Although the hereditary variables that contribute to bladder cancer are poorly understood, there is some evidence to suggest that a family history of the disease increases the risk.

**8.** Bladder cancer incidence differs by race and ethnicity. It affects more Caucasians than African-Americans or Hispanics, for instance.

**9.** Bladder cancer incidence varies by region, with some places having greater rates than others because of environmental and lifestyle variables.

**10.** There may be a small increase in the risk of acquiring bladder cancer as a secondary cancer after receiving chemotherapy or radiation therapy for another type of cancer.

Having one or more of these risk factors does not ensure that bladder cancer will develop; people without any of these risk factors can still get the disease. Many people who are at risk for bladder cancer never actually get it. These factors often interact in subtle ways, making it difficult to pinpoint a single cause for bladder cancer. Prevention and better outcomes are possible through regular checkups, early detection, and changes in lifestyle, such as stopping smoking. A medical professional should be consulted if there is any uncertainty about one's risk of developing bladder cancer.

# CHAPTER TWO
## How to Recognize It and What It Is

There is a wide range of symptoms associated with bladder cancer, and the disease is normally diagnosed with a battery of examinations. The most common symptoms, tests, and procedures used to diagnose bladder cancer are as follows:

**What to Look For:**

**1.** Blood in the urine (hematuria) is the primary symptom of bladder cancer and typically the first indicator. This may make the urine seem pink, crimson, or brown. The blood in your urine may come and go in spurts.

**2.** Urinating Frequently Even When the Bladder Isn't Full: People with bladder cancer may have an increased urgency to urinate and an increased frequency of urine.

**3.** Discomfort or a Burning feeling: Pain or a burning feeling may be experienced while urinating.

**4.** Discomfort in the Lower Back or Pelvis Bladder cancer has been linked to discomfort in the perineum (the area between the scrotum and the anus in men) and the lower back.

**5.** Changes in Urinary Routine Difficulty urinating, a weak urine stream, or an incomplete emptying of the bladder are all examples of urinary routine changes.

**6.** Unexpected Weight Loss and Exhaustion: These symptoms may occur in the later stages of bladder cancer.

## Methods of Diagnosis:

**1.** A urinalysis is a simple test for the urinary tract that might reveal the presence of blood, abnormal cells, and other warning signs.

**2.** Through the urethra, a cystoscope (a thin, flexible tube with a camera at its tip) is put into the bladder to examine its interior. The doctor is then able to examine the bladder's inner lining and check for tumors or other abnormalities thanks to this visualization.

**3.** If abnormal areas are detected after a cystoscopy, a biopsy of the bladder lining may be performed. The presence of cancer cells is then confirmed by examining the biopsy under a microscope.

**4.** Computed tomography (CT) scans, magnetic resonance imaging (MRI), and ultrasound are all examples of imaging procedures that can be used to determine how far the cancer has spread and if it has spread beyond the bladder wall and adjacent lymph nodes. With the results of these exams, the cancer can be staged more accurately.

**5.** Urography, also known as an intravenous pyelogram (IVP) or retrograde pyelogram (RP), is a special kind of X-ray that allows doctors to see the urinary tract and see any abnormalities.

**6. Cytology of the Urine:** A test for bladder cancer that looks for abnormal cells in a urine sample.

**7. Biological Markers:** Urine testing that looks for certain proteins or genetic markers can help doctors diagnose and track bladder cancer.

When used together, these diagnostic tools allow doctors to confirm the presence of bladder cancer, assess the disease's stage, and devise a treatment strategy. Earlier diagnosis is crucial since it increases the likelihood of a positive outcome from treatment. Urgent medical attention is warranted if you or a loved one are experiencing any of the warning signs associated with bladder cancer.

# CHAPTER THREE
## Alternative Treatments

Treatment options for bladder cancer vary from patient to patient based on a number of characteristics such as cancer kind, stage, general health, and personal preference. The standard methods for dealing with bladder cancer are as follows:

## 1. Surgery:

• Transurethral resection of bladder tumor (TURBT): a cystoscope can be used to remove a bladder tumor in its early stages. This is a minimally invasive technique, meaning that no incisions will be made on the skin.

• When the bladder cancer has spread into the bladder muscle wall or when the cancer is of a high grade, a partial or radical cystectomy may be necessary. In more severe situations, other organs and lymph nodes may also need to be removed along with the bladder during a radical cystectomy.

• After a radical cystectomy, a new system must be developed to collect and flush the patient's urine. This can be performed by different surgical methods, including ileal conduit (urine drains through a stoma), continent cutaneous reservoir (uses a pouch to store urine), or neobladder reconstruction (creates a new bladder-like reservoir).

## 2. Intravenous Treatment:

• Bacillus Calmette-Guérin (BCG): BCG is an immunotherapy method that involves injecting a diluted strain of the tuberculosis bacterium into the bladder. The immune system is prompted into action against cancer cells.

**3. Radiotherapy, or Radiation Treatment:**

• High-powered X-rays are focused on the bladder to kill cancer cells, a process known as external beam radiation therapy. It is frequently used in conjunction with surgical procedures, and in the absence of those, as a main treatment.

• **Internal Radiation (Brachytherapy):** Radioactive materials are implanted inside or near the tumor in the bladder to provide radiation directly to the cancer cells.

## 4. Chemotherapy:

- **Intravesical Chemotherapy:** Chemotherapy medications are given directly into the bladder via a catheter. To prevent cancer from returning after surgery, this is often prescribed.

More advanced or metastatic bladder cancer can be treated with chemotherapy medicines that are administered systemically, either intravenously or orally. Cancer that has progressed beyond the bladder frequently requires this treatment.

## 5. Immunotherapy:

• Drugs like pembrolizumab and atezolizumab operate by blocking particular proteins that allow cancer cells to elude the immune system. In cases of advanced or metastatic bladder cancer, these medications are prescribed.

## 6. Therapeutic Aiming:

• Erdafitinib and enfortumab vedotin are examples of targeted medications that attack cancer development at a molecular level. They treat advanced bladder cancer caused by certain mutations.

**7.** Clinical trials Patients who enroll in these studies may have the opportunity to receive experimental treatments before they are made generally available to the public. New medications, treatment methods, and even therapeutic synergies can all be tested in clinical trials.

Cancer staging informs treatment decisions. Surgery is the mainstay treatment for patients with early-stage bladder cancer, but other methods, such as chemotherapy, radiation therapy, immunotherapy, or targeted therapy, may need to be combined to treat patients with more advanced or metastatic disease. Each patient's course of treatment is developed individually, taking into account their unique medical history and the advice of their healthcare providers. Treatment choices and potential side effects for bladder cancer should be discussed with a healthcare provider before making any final decisions.

## How to Handle a Medical Prognosis and Treatment

Treatment for bladder cancer, if diagnosed, can be taxing both mentally and physically. There are both tangible and intangible factors to adjusting to a diagnosis and subsequent therapy. To aid individuals and their loved ones on this challenging path, here are some strategies and tips:

## 1. Ask for Help:

• If you need someone to talk to, call, or text a loved one. Having somebody you can lean on during this time can be invaluable.

• Think about connecting with others through a bladder cancer support group or forum. Connecting with others who are experiencing or have had similar difficulties can help you feel less alone.

## 2. Get some training:

• Get educated on bladder cancer, your options for care, and what to anticipate. Understanding the disease and its management can lessen anxiety and help you make educated decisions.

## 3. Talk to Your Medical Staff:

• Keep an open line of contact with your healthcare providers at all times. Inquire and voice your worries. You may rely on the assistance and direction of your healthcare professionals throughout your treatment.

## 4. Stress Management:

• To lessen the emotional toll of a diagnosis and subsequent therapy, try deep breathing exercises, meditation, yoga, or mindfulness.

## 5. Diet and Physical Activity:

• Eat healthily to promote healing and general well-being. If you feel the need, talk to a dietician or nutritionist.

• If your health permits you, maintain as much physical activity as possible.

## 6. Treatment of Adverse Events:

• Think ahead about the treatment's probable negative effects and figure out a plan with your medical staff to deal with them. Medications and alterations to one's way of life are frequently helpful.

## 7. Be Your Own Best Advocate:

• It is your right to have a say in how your health care is provided. If you have problems or preferences, don't hesitate to share them.

## 8. Keep an Eye on Your Mood:

Maintain vigilance on your mental health. It's normal to experience a range of emotions, including dread, anxiety, and sadness. Talking to a counselor or mental health professional may help if these emotions become too much to handle.

## 9. Maintain a Diary:

• The act of putting pen to paper can be quite healing. You can use it to keep tabs on your symptoms and how well your treatment is working.

## 10. Keep a Regular Schedule:

• Maintaining a regular pattern can be comforting in times of change and instability.

## 11. Arrange Your Future:

• You and your healthcare team should talk about your goals for the future. The prognosis and treatment's potential long-term implications can be discussed with them.

## 12. Rely on Friends and Family

• Your loved ones may also benefit from counseling after hearing the news of your illness. Encourage open interactions with them, and consider incorporating them in your treatment as appropriate.

## 13. Prioritize Happiness:

• Despite the significance of treatment, it is essential to put quality of life first. Share your values and preferences for treatment with your healthcare team.

## 14. Check Out Non-Conventional Treatments:

• Acupuncture, massage, and herbal supplements are just a few examples of complementary and alternative therapies that have been shown to be beneficial in alleviating symptoms and side effects for some patients.

It's important to find the methods of dealing with bladder cancer that work best for you, as each person's experience is different. Your healthcare team, together with assistance from friends and family, can be essential resources as you navigate this tough journey.

# CHAPTER FOUR
## Methods to Reduce the Risk of Bladder Cancer

Although it is not always practicable, there are several things you may do to lessen your chances of developing bladder cancer. Advice for avoiding bladder cancer:

**1.** To reduce your chance of bladder cancer, you should stop smoking. The best thing you can do to lower your risk is to stop smoking. Stay away from smokers, both active and passive.

**2.** To reduce the risk of developing bladder cancer, workers should take all necessary precautions when exposed on the job to chemicals such aromatic amines and polycyclic aromatic hydrocarbons. Protect yourself from toxic chemicals by wearing protective gear.

**3.** Keep yourself hydrated by consuming lots of water. Staying well-hydrated may help dilute potentially toxic compounds in the urine and lessen the risk of bladder discomfort. The average adult needs about 8 cups of water per day (64 ounces), but this might vary widely.

**4. Eat Healthily:** Vitamins and antioxidants included in a diet high in fruits and vegetables may reduce cancer risk if consumed on a regular basis. A lower risk of bladder cancer has been linked to diets rich in fruits and vegetables.

**5.** Maintaining a healthy weight and good health in general can be aided by an active lifestyle. According to recommendations, adults should engage in at least 150 minutes of moderate-intensity aerobic activity per week, or 75 minutes of vigorous-intensity aerobic activity per week.

**6.** As long-term exposure to arsenic has been associated to an increased risk of bladder cancer, it is important to be wary of ingesting water and food sources that may contain high quantities of this toxin.

**7. Practice Safe Sex:** Some research have revealed a potential association between certain sexually transmitted illnesses and an increased risk of bladder cancer. Safe sexual behavior and timely medical attention for infections may help lower this danger.

**8.** Although there is no evidence linking alcohol to an increased risk of bladder cancer, excessive alcohol use is harmful to health in general and should be avoided. If you drink alcohol, do it in moderation.

**9.** If you have a family history of bladder cancer or other risk factors for the disease, it is recommended that you consider the potential of regular checkups with your healthcare professional. For those with a higher risk, early diagnosis and treatment can be lifesaving.

**10.** Educate yourself about the symptoms of bladder cancer, which include blood in the urine, a need to urinate frequently, and pain while urinating. Get checked out right away if you experience any strange symptoms.

These measures can help reduce your risk of developing bladder cancer, but they are not a failsafe against the disease. Even if there are no obvious risk factors, anyone can develop bladder cancer. Managing bladder cancer and improving treatment outcomes depend on regular checkups and early identification. Get in touch with a doctor if you have questions regarding your individual risk for bladder cancer.

## Conclusion

Bladder cancer is a multifaceted illness with a wide range of possible causes and treatments. While the exact causes of bladder cancer may not always be evident, there are activities individuals may do to lower their risk, such as quitting smoking, reducing chemical exposures, and maintaining a healthy lifestyle. Early identification and diagnosis play a significant role in improving treatment outcomes, so it's essential to be aware of the common signs and symptoms of bladder cancer and seek fast medical assistance if necessary.

Surgery, chemotherapy, radiation treatment, immunotherapy, or targeted therapy may be used to treat bladder cancer, however these methods vary greatly depending on the cancer's kind and stage. Seeking out community, keeping up on treatment developments, controlling stress, and prioritizing wellness are all important aspects of the emotional and practical work of coping with a diagnosis of bladder cancer and its treatment.

It is important to work closely with healthcare specialists to create a specialized treatment plan for your bladder cancer, as each person's experience is different. In spite of the difficulties associated with bladder cancer, you can face them head-on if you take preventative measures, monitor your health closely, and enlist the help of loved ones and professionals.

**THE END**